Lamine Ghanem Lakhal

# ECHOCARDIOGRAPHY IN THE EMERGENCY DEPARTMENT

Lamine Ghanem Lakhal

# ECHOCARDIOGRAPHY IN THE EMERGENCY DEPARTMENT

ScienciaScripts

**Imprint**



Cover image: www.ingimage.com

This book is a translation from the original published under ISBN 978-620-6-73035-4.

Publisher:
Sciencia Scripts
is a trademark of
Dodo Books Indian Ocean Ltd. and OmniScriptum S.R.L publishing group

120 High Road, East Finchley, London, N2 9ED, United Kingdom
Str. Armeneasca 28/1, office 1, Chisinau MD-2012, Republic of Moldova, Europe
Managing Directors: Ieva Konstantinova, Victoria Ursu
info@omniscriptum.com

Printed at: see last page
**ISBN: 978-620-8-64262-4**

***ECHOCARDIOGRAPHY IN THE EMERGENCY DEPARTMENT***

***DR GHANEM LAKHAL LAMINE***

## TABLE OF CONTENTS

# 1. INTRODUCTION

Transthoracic echocardiography in the emergency department and intensive care unit provides answers to a number of classic questions frequently asked by practitioners working in these departments.

Echocardiography is a powerful diagnostic tool if the usual steps medical reasoning are followed: history-taking and clinical examination.

This is a "targeted" examination designed to provide easy answers to simple clinical questions:

Does the patient require volume expansion or not?

"Assessment of blood volume

Does the patient require Dobutamine support?

"Assessment of systolic function

Is the patient in respiratory distress due to PAO or pulmonary infection?

"Evaluation of LV filling pressures

All these questions, together with a systematic search pericardial fluid effusion or pleural fluid or gas effusion, need to be answered quickly and clearly in order to guide the therapeutic management of these patients.

# 2. ECHOCARDIOGRAPHIC EVALUATION OF SYSTOLIC FUNCTION

## 2.1 ASSESSMENT

The best assessment of systolic LV function is visual. It requires an expert, trained operator, with an eye that is used to combining numerical assessment by ejection fraction or shortening fraction with visual assessment of the quality of contraction.

In emergency and intensive care , this assessment is straightforward:

- Preserved systolic function corresponds to an ejection fraction of over 50%.
- Moderate LV dysfunction corresponds to an ejection fraction of between 35 and 45%.
- Severe systolic LV dysfunction corresponds to an ejection fraction less than 25%.

The quality of contraction must be assessed in several planes and in both longitudinal and transverse axes.

## 2.2 ASSESSMENT

Unlike segmental assessment, global assessment provides a better assessment of ventricular function. The two most commonly used methods are: calculation of the ejection fraction using the SIMPSON method, and measurement of aortic flow using a calculation of sub-aortic VTI. [1]

### *2.2.1* CALCULATION THE EJECTION FRACTION

The calculation is simple: measure the initial volume in diastole, then the terminal volume after emptying at the end of systole, and calculate the ejection fraction using the formula: [2].

**FE = VTD-VTS/VTD**

This method is validated regardless of LV geometry, and with or without the presence of dyssynchronisation.

Examples of dyssynchronisation: LBBB, ACFA, kinetic disorders, paradoxical septum

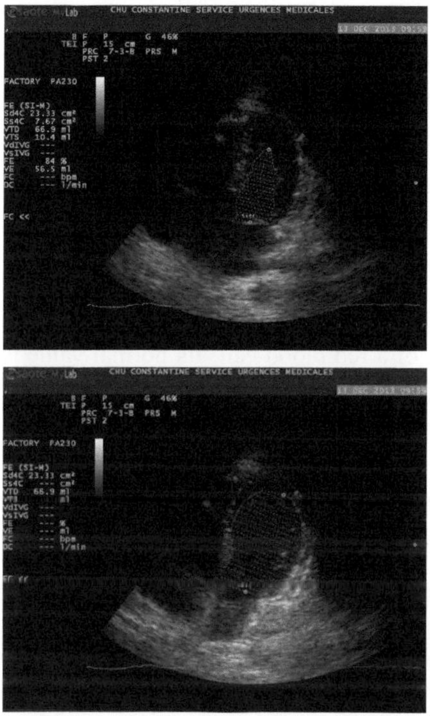


Figure 1: Ventricular volumes in systole and diastole[2]

The problem with the disc method is the difficulty in detecting the contours of the endocardium, which requires training and experience. This detection can be facilitated by the injection of a contrast agent [3]

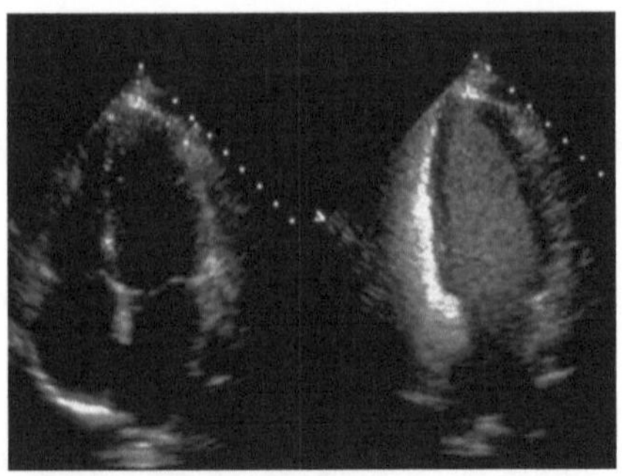

Figure 2: Echocardiography with intraventricular contrast medium

### *2.2.2* CALCULATION ITV UNDER AORTIC

The sub-aortic time-velocity integral, known as the sub-aortic VTI, represents the ejection distance of a red blood cell. Its normal value is 20 cm, corresponds to an ejection capacity (ejection distance) for the left ventricle of 20 cm. This calculation is based on a three- or five-cavity apical slice, the pulsed Doppler shot placed under the aortic sigmoid, with an appropriate sampling window.The measurement is displayed with the aortic ejection curve plotted

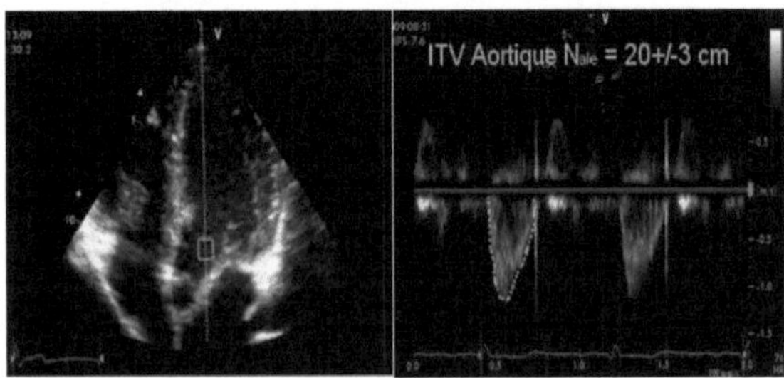


Figure 3: Calculation sub-aortic VTI

Aortic flow is calculated using the formula: AORTIC FLOW= ITV X FC X AORTIC SURFACE

## 2.3 EVALUATION SEGMENTS

Several methods are used for segmental assessment of ventricular function. It should be noted that indices using segmental assessment are only validated in patients with good contraction harmony (synchronisation) between the four cavities. [4][5]

### *2.3.1* MEASUREMENT OF THE FRACTION OF SHORTENING

This is the technique most commonly used by cardiologists. It is quick and easy to perform, and gives a figure known as the shortening fraction (SF). It is measured from a long axis parasterenal section, respecting a line which must be perpendicular to the different walls:

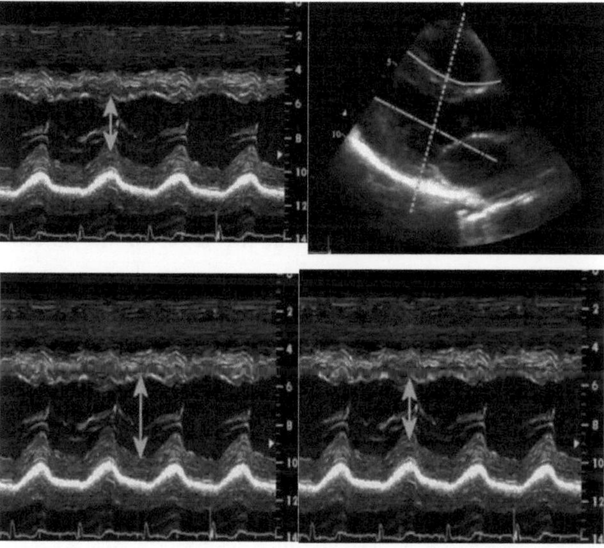

Figure 4: Measurement of shortening fraction

The shortening fraction is calculated using a simple formula based on the diameter at telediastole and telesystole.

FR= DTD -DTS /DTD Normale 37+/- 8% (normal)

The ejection can be calculated from the same formula, by deducting the volume from the diameter using the Teicholz formula

**V (ml)= $7D^3/2.4+D$**

**Technique not valid if :**

**LBBB, paradoxical septum, kinetic disorders, WPW**

### *2.3.2* MEASUREMENT OF THE VELOCITY OF MOVEMENT OF THE LATERAL MITRAL ANNULUS USING TISSUE DOPPLER

Tissue Doppler measures the speed of displacement of a myocardial wall. Based on this principle, measuring the displacement of the lateral ring of the mitral valve during systole enables us to assess the quality of contractility, and therefore systolic function.This measurement is taken from a four-cavity apical slice. The tissue Doppler shot is placed at the level of the lateral ring of the mitral valve, giving the following appearance;[5]

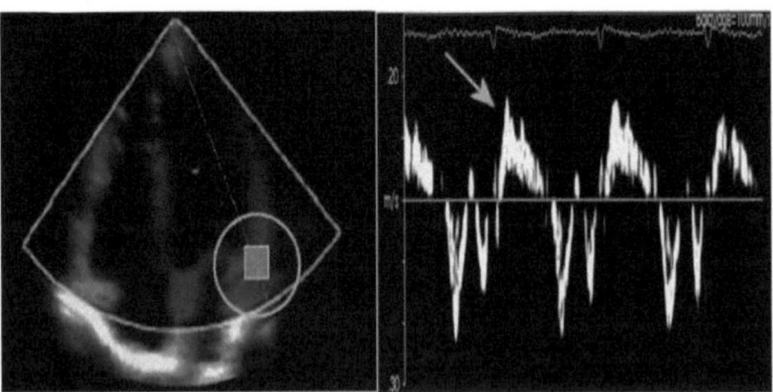

Figure 5: Tissue Doppler in lateral ring of the mitral valve

The positive wave in systole is called the Sa wave. Its normal value is equal to 10.3 +/- 1.4 cm/s. The ejection fraction is considered to be less than 50% if the

Sa speed is less than 08 cm/s.This quick and simple technique is not valid in the presence of dyssynchronisation.

### *2.3.3* MEASUREMENT OF THE DISPLACEMENT DISTANCE OF THE LATERAL MITRAL ANNULUS USING TISSUE DOPPLER

Measurement of the displacement distance of the lateral mitral annulus is a method of assessing the quality of systolic function, known as MAPSE or mitral valve lateral annulus excursion.a four-cavity apical section, the TM line is placed at the level of the lateral ring, giving the following appearance: [5]

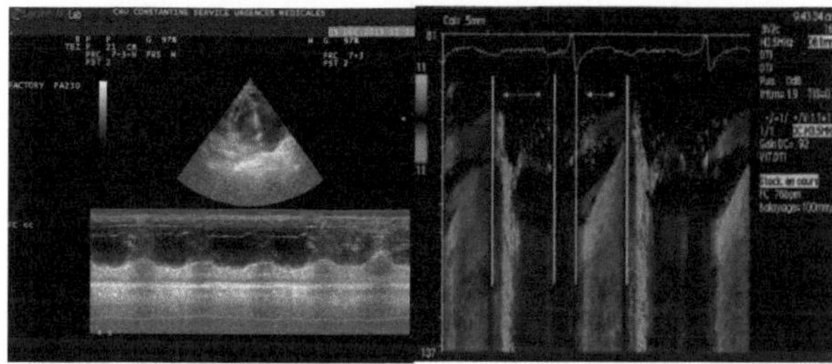

Figure 6: MAPSE mitral lateral annulus displacement distance

The normal displacement distance is equal to 15 mm The ejection considered to be less than 50% if this MAPSE distance is less than 10 mm. This method is not valid in cases of dyssynchronisation.

## 2.4 SUMMARY

Global assessment should always be preferred to segmental ones. Because of the LV geometry, it is not possible to estimate an ejection fraction or shortening for the right ventricle. Assessment of LV systolic function uses TAPSE and pulmonary VTI.Ventricular function is best assessed visually.

# 3. ECHOCARDIOGRAPHIC EVALUATION OF DIASTOLIC FUNCTION

## 3.1 REMINDER PHYSIOLOGY

Diastolic function is schematically separated into two phases: the relaxation phase and the compliance phase [6].

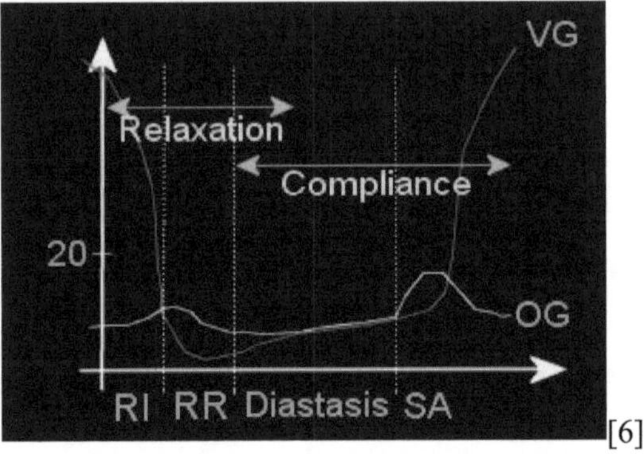

[6]

Figure 7: Physiology of the diastolic phase

Relaxation is an active phase which takes place with the atrioventricular and sigmoid valves closed. Its aim is to reduce intra-ventricular pressure to allow the atrioventricular valves to open. Compliance is a passive phase, which begins after opening of the atrioventricular septal defects and the start of rapid filling. The change in ventricular volume occurs under the effect of filling, and depends on the compliance of the myocardial wall.

Once the filling process has begun, the three classic phases take place:

- Rapid ventricular filling
- The diastasis phase of pressure equalisation

• Active filling by atrial contraction

Diastolic function is assessed by measuring OG-VG ventricular filling velocities for the left heart.This is measured by pulsed Doppler at the coaptation point of the large and small mitral valves.

## 3.2 MITRAL PROFILE

The mitral profile is a term used in everyday practice to give an idea of left ventricular filling pressures. It is the expression of variations in filling velocities in proto- and telediastole.

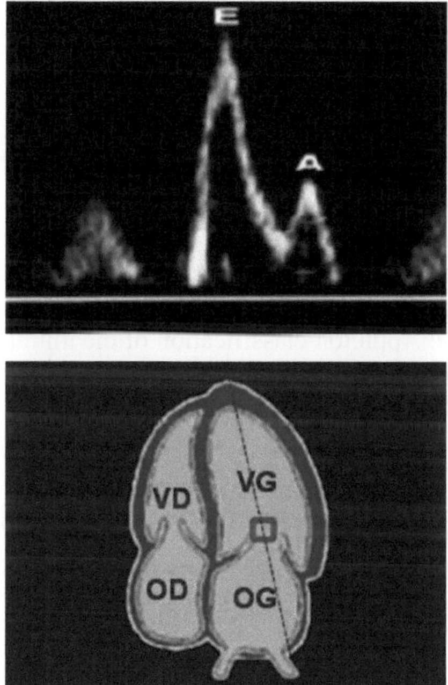


Figure 8: Mitral profile

This profile is formed by two waves: the E wave (EARLY) is the rate of rapid ventricular filling, and the A wave (ATRIUM) represents the rate of active atrial filling.The so-called mitral profile is determined by the E/A ratio.

## 3.3 THE DIFFERENT TYPES OF MITRAL PROFILE

The normal E/A ratio is between 1 and 2. A ratio greater than 2 a compliance disorder and a probable increase in left filling pressures. A ratio of less than 1 is called a relaxation disorder, eliminates the increase in filling pressures and is physiological from a certain age[7].

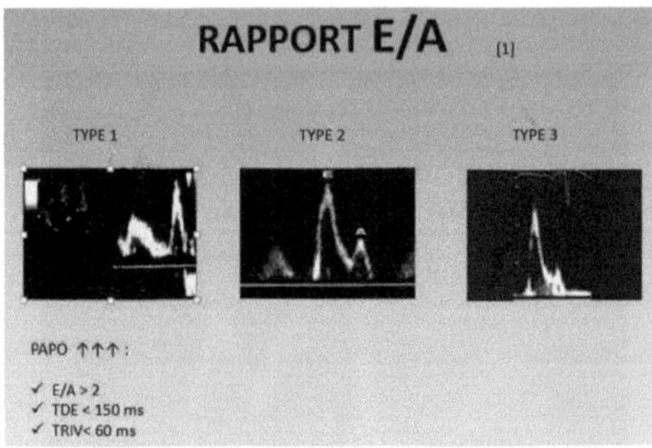


Figure 9: Appleton classification of the mitral profile

**The type 1 profile** is known as relaxation disorder. Filling pressures are normal

**The type 2 profile** is called the normal profile in young subjects. It is pathological in elderly subjects, in which case it is called "normalised". The normalised profile is due to an increase in filling pressures.

**The type 3 profile** is always pathological, and probably indicates an increase filling pressures.

### 3.4 DTI TISSUE DOPPLER MEASUREMENT

Tissue Doppler is used to measure the speed of movement a ventricular wall. The flow velocity of the liquid (blood), called v1, causes the myocardial wall to move with another velocity called v2.The v1/v2 ratio expresses the quality of compliance of the myocardial wall. The higher the ratio, the less compliant the wall. Based on the same principle, LV compliance is assessed by the E/Ea ratio, where E blood flow velocity and Ea represents myocardial wall displacement velocity. [8] High left filling pressures if the E/Ea ratio is greater than 14.

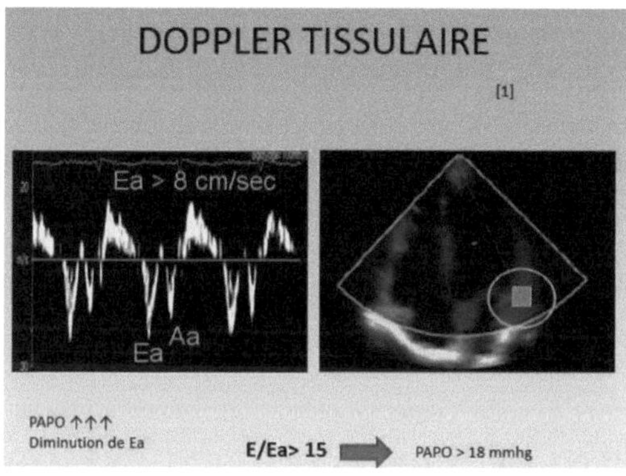


Figure 10: Evaluation of filling pressures using the E/Ea ratio

### 3.5 MEASUREMENT OF PROPAGATION VELOCITY IN DIASTOLE

In cases of increased left filling pressures, there is an increase in filling velocities only in protodiastole. However, the average of these velocity variations over entire duration of diastole is reduced because of the alteration in the LV-OG gradient [9].

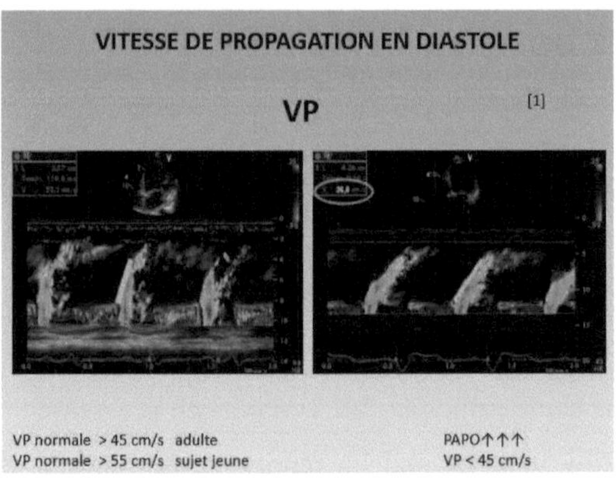


Figure 11: Velocity of flow propagation in diastole

This velocity is measured by calculating the opening slope of the large mitral valve in diastole, by combining colour Doppler and TM mode. Filling pressures are considered high when the PV is less than 45 cm/s.It is an index that depends little on myocardial load conditions (preload and afterload).

### 3.6 MEASUREMENT OF PULMONARY VENOUS FLOW

**This** method is used assess left filling pressures when previous methods are inconclusive. The Doppler shot is placed the level of pulmonary vein-left atrium junction. The negative flow alone determines what is known as the pulmonary A wave [10].

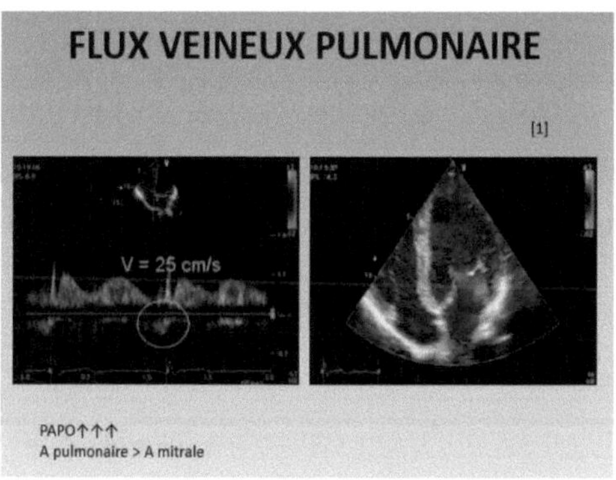


Figure 12: Pulmonary venous flow

Left filling pressures are considered high if the pulmonary A wave is greater than mitral flow A wave in duration and amplitude.

## 3.7 COMBINED INDICES

Combination of different indices is important for a reliable assessment filling pressures

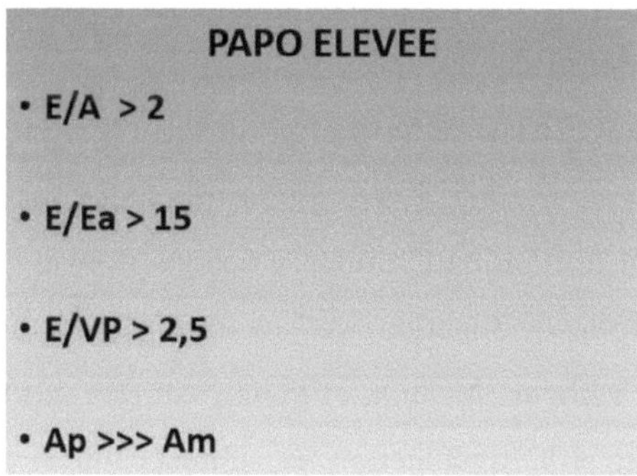


Figure 13: Combined indices assessing filling pressures

These combined indices use four parameters: filling velocity in protodiastole **E**, wall displacement velocity in protodiastole **Ea**, mean propagation velocity in diastole **VP**, and pulmonary venous flow **FVP.**

### 3.8 SUMMARY

In practical terms, the diagram below represents the classic method of LV filling pressures. Left atrial size and IT leak rate were not included in the diagram[11].

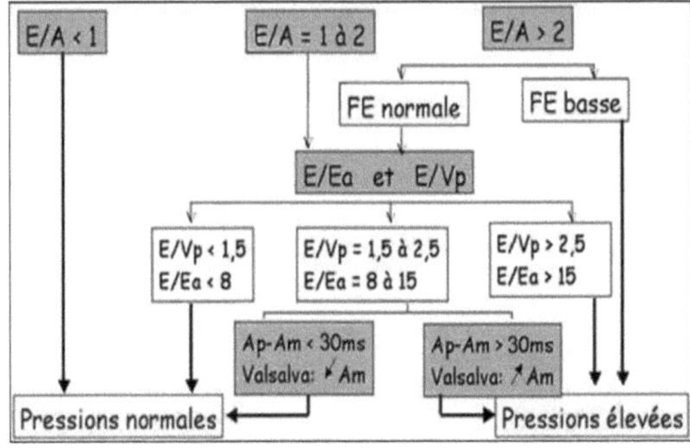


Figure 14: Summary of filling pressure assessment [11].

What is currently used are the ESC recommendations based on the study of the mitral profile, LV compliance by the E/Ea ratio, the size of the left atrium and the tricuspid leak rate[12].The main finding in the ESC diagram is the lack of use of E-wave deceleration time, a very interesting index for assessing pressures in patients with atrial fibrillation.Pulmonary venous flow and S/D ratio are used in cases of LV systolic dysfunction, and to detect early diastolic dysfunction (elevation of LVOT without elevation of POG). An E/A ratio greater than 2 in a patient with systolic LV dysfunction is almost 100% equivalent to high POG.Comparing the A wave of the pulmonary venous flow with the A wave of the mitral profile allows early detection of an increase in LV filling pressures. IT leak rate is statistically well correlated PCP (pulmonary capillary wedge pressure).

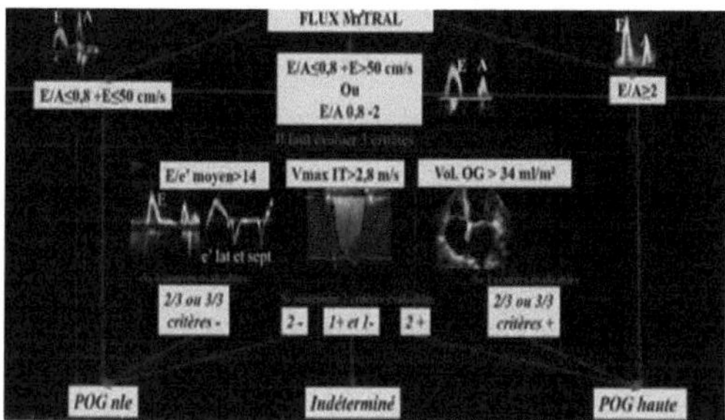


Figure 15: Assessment of filling pressures (ESC recommendations)

# 4. NON-INVASIVE ASSESSMENT OF FLUTTER IN A PATIENT WITH HEMODYNAMIC INSTABILITY

Faced with any haemodynamic instability, the clinician will ask the classic questions: Should I fill or not? and what index should I use to assess blood volume?In the absence of available monitoring, he will use clinical parameters to guide his volemic expansion. The clinical parameters often used are the context haemodynamic instability and the filling status of the jugular veins [13]

## 4.1 THE CLINICAL CONTEXT

Assessment of the clinical context is the first step towards a practical approach blood volume status. A young patient, the victim of a road traffic accident, with pale mucous membranes and skin, is likely to be in hypovolaemic shock due to haemorrhage. An infant presenting with shock and diarrhoea is likely to be hypovolaemic. Haemodynamic instability in a patient with a history of dilated cardiomyopathy is probably not hypovolaemic[14]. The presence of a clinical context of hypovolaemia is a sufficient argument to start vascular filling without waiting for other methods blood volume to be used.

## 4.2 CLINICAL FILLING OF THE EXTERNAL JUGULAR VEINS

The filling of the external jugular veins is an important factor to consider when assessing blood volume. Well-filled external jugular veins are an argument for high right filling pressures in the right heart chambers, and the shock is probably not hypovolaemic in origin.Flat jugular veins in a patient in circulatory failure is sufficient evidence for the diagnosis of hypovolaemic shock, and for low right filling pressures allowing volaemic expansion.

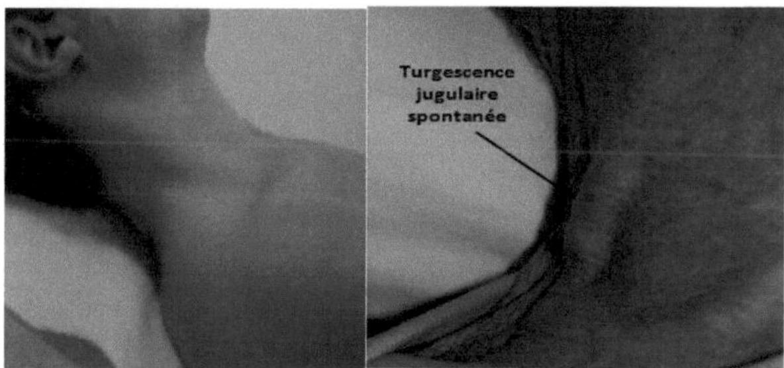


Figure 16: Assessment of right filling pressures based on the diameter of the external jugular veins

If the clinical situation is , the practitioner should use both static and dynamic indices to assess blood volume.Static indices are based on measurement of left and right filling pressures (PVC and PAPO), and on the measurement of the volumes of the two ventricles or the vascular venous trunks (the two vena cava). These static indices are informative only in their extreme values. Very low CVP and PAPO levels may volume expansion without guaranteeing response to filling (increased cardiac output)The same applies to cavity volumes, ventricular volumes are a likely argument for hypovolaemia without guaranteeing response to filling. [15]

## 4.3 THE VOLUME OF THE VENTRICULAR CAVITIES

The volume of the ventricular cavities assessed by echocardiography is a static element to be taken into account when assessing blood volume. A dilated left ventricle, or one with a volume in excess of 80 ml/surface area, is indicative of high or normal filling pressures. Shock is probably not hypovolaemic.

An empty left ventricle will have a reduced volume, leading in most to systolic ventricular exclusion, which is a major sign of hypovolaemia.A small right ventricle normal or low right filling pressures. An LV/DV ratio > or equal to 1 probably indicates against any volume expansion.

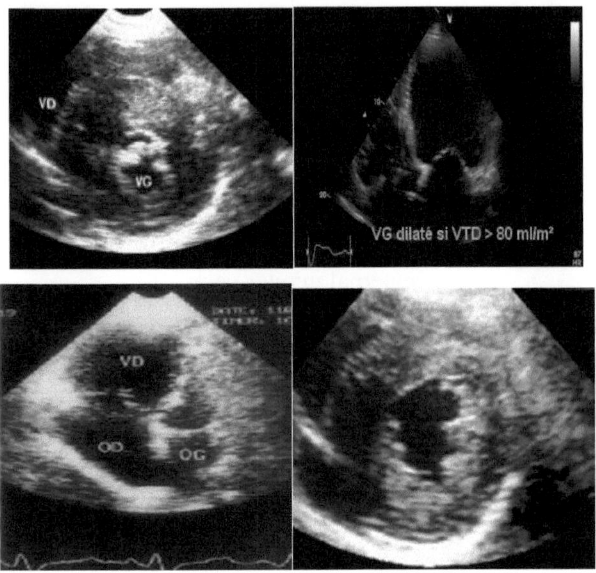


Figure 17: Assessment of blood volume based on cavity volumes

## 4.4 AN ASSESSMENT OF VENTRICULAR FILLING PRESSURES

Assessment of the two ventricular filling pressures (right and left) is used guide fluid intake.High right and/or left filling pressures are contraindications any volume expansion. Assessment of left filling pressures by echocardiography involves the use of the classic parameters; E/Ea ratio, left atrial size, and tricuspid leak rate (see chapter on assessment of LV filling pressures)[12]. Right filling pressures are assessed by evaluating the compliance of the vena cava by measuring variations in its diameter between inspiratory and expiratory times.

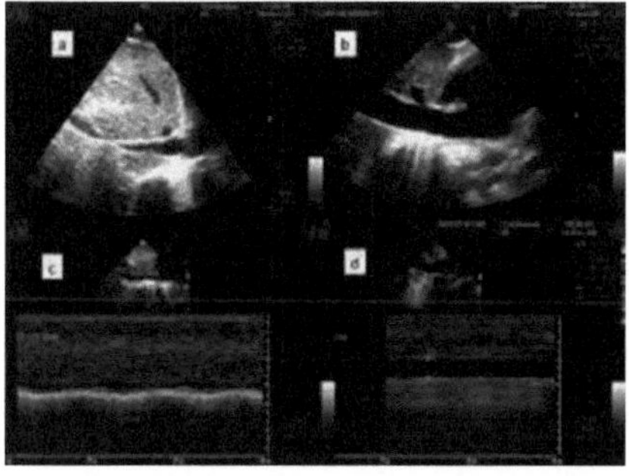

Figure 18: Study inferior vena cava compliance

## 4.5 DYNAMIC EVALUATION OF VARIATIONS IN THE DIAMETER OF VCI

key to interpreting dynamic variations in the diameter of the inferior vena cava is the clinical context[16]. A flat vena cava is not synonymous with hypovolaemia. A flat vena cava is indicative low filling pressures in the right cavities, which are generally physiological in an unshocked subject. A flat vena cava can only used to initiate volume expansion in patients circulatory failure or in patients with ARF, in order to restore diuresis. The diameter of the IVC during inspiration or expiration is not important. What is important is the variation of this diameter in relation to the mean value, expressing what is known as the compliance of the IVC. The study of venous compliance is a dynamic parameter which evaluates a static pressure, the PVC. Cellular compliance alone cannot predict the response to filling and preload-dependence states. The best parameters assessing blood volume are dynamic parameters, which assess the variation in cardiac output between inspiratory and expiratory times. Cardiac output can be assessed using a number of non-invasive indices, the most widely used of which is sub-aortic VTI.

## 4.6 PRINCIPLE OF DYNAMIC INDICES

The assessment of blood volume using dynamic indices is based on the interpretation of cyclic variations in cardiac output between inspiratory and expiratory times [17]

Heart-lung interaction and cyclic variations in myocardial load conditions (preload and afterload) lead to cyclic variations in cardiac output. Patients are labelled hypovolaemic if variations in cardiac output exceed a certain percentage of the mean, depending on the method used to calculate cardiac output.

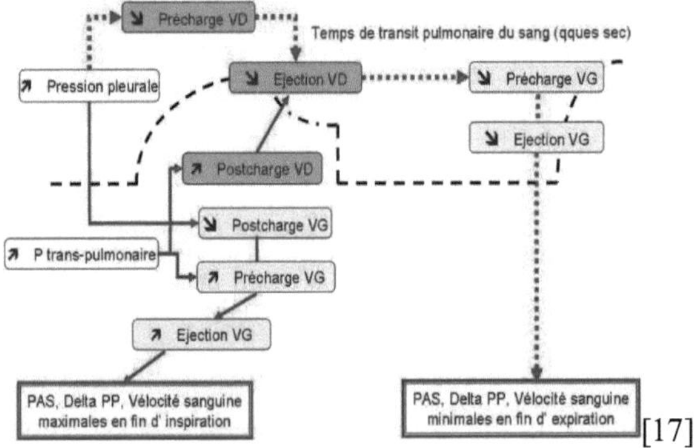


[17]

Figure 19: Heart-lung interaction ventilated patients

## 4.7 VARIATIONS ITV UNDER AORTIC

The time-velocity integral known as sub-aortic VTI is an indirect expression of cardiac output. It provides indirect information on the quality of ventricular systolic function by measuring the ejection distance of a red blood cell, which averages 20 cm. Cardiac output= ITV X heart rate X aortic surface area Physiologically, there is a variation in left ventricular stroke caused by variations in ventricular load conditions (preload and afterload) between inspiration and expiration. You have to accept variations in cardiac output that do not exceed a certain threshold.

The accentuation of variations in cardiac output between the two respiratory times is an argument for hypovolaemia. Several methods are used to assess the variation in cardiac output. The change subaortic VTI between inspiration and expiration is a classic method used to assess blood volume [18]

Apart from passive leg raising, all the techniques used have only been validated in ventilated patients who are well adapted to the ventilator.

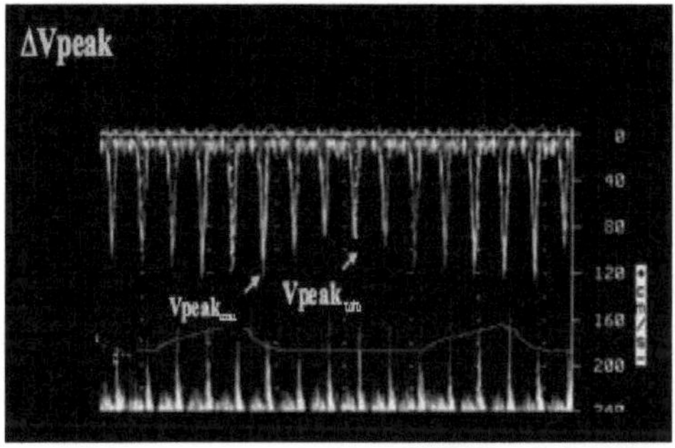


Figure 20: Variations in subaortic VTI (oesophageal Doppler)

Variation of subaortic VTI can be used in several situations:

- The fill test
- The LJP (passive leg raising manoeuvre)

**IMPORTANT+++**

**The criterion for continued filling should always be cardiac output and not arterial pressure.**

**Discontinuation of volemic expansion may be based solely on changes in cardiac output or on clinical criteria (improvement in signs circulatory**

**failure).**

**Patients with high left or right filling pressures should not be filled.**

## 4.8 PRACTICAL ASSESSMENT OF FLUTTER BY ECHOCARDIOGRAPHY

The use of echocardiography enables a static assessment blood volume, volumes and surface areas, and filling pressures which can be deduced from the mitral profile and through a study of ventricular compliance using tissue Doppler. By coupling systolic and diastolic functions, the patient can be positioned on Frank Starling curve. The use of cell compliance and filling tests is proposed in grey zone situations [19].

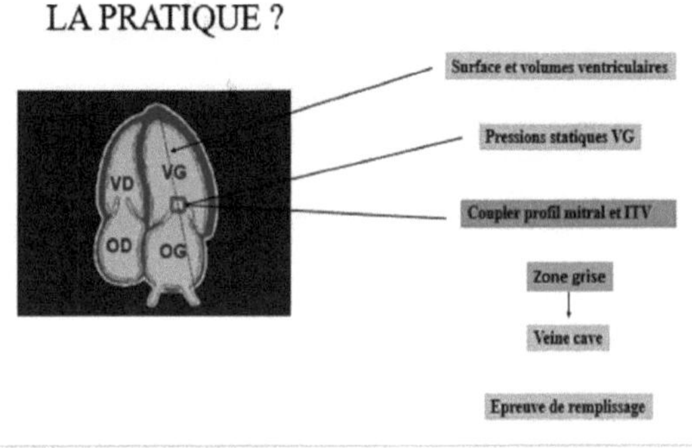


Figure 21: Use of echocardiography assess blood volume

Combining an assessment of diastolic function (E/A ratio) with that of systolic function (subaortic VTI) makes it possible, above all, to position the patient's volume status on the Frank Starling curve.

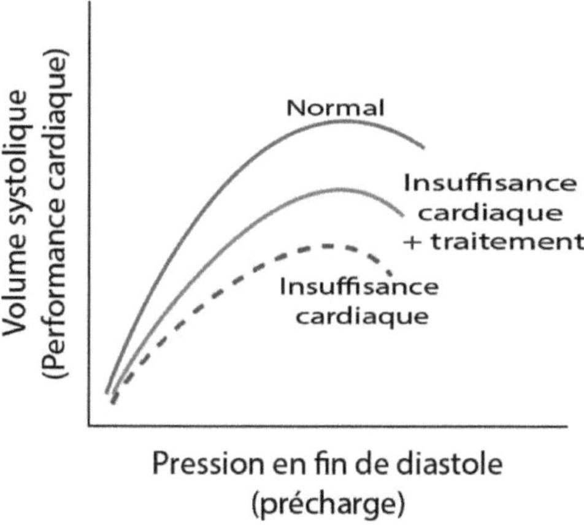


Figure 22: Frank Starling curve

Poor preload reserve is a classic feature of patients with systolic ventricular dysfunction,There are three possible situations:The first combines low filling pressures with a collapsed cardiac output (the patient is clearly preload dependent).The second situation is different depending on the pre-load reserve:In a healthy heart, the preload-dependent part is always present, with a VTI between 10 and 15, and volume expansion can increase cardiac output. In a patient with a poor preload reserve, the patient is in the plateau phase, and the risk of overload is high. The last situation will involve high left filling pressures with a VTI greater than 20 cm (filling risks flooding the lung and all volume expansion must be stopped). Often, when we are in a grey zone and the various indices are inconclusive, we are obliged to use the filling test to label preload-dependent subjects (subjects who are able to increase their cardiac output with volume expansion).

Two methods are proposed:

**Mini-fill test**: 1.4 ml/kg over one minute and see change in ITV Or

**Graduated filling test**: 4ml/kg of fluids, with continuous monitoring of sub-aortic ITV variation

The proposed scheme guiding volume expansion in a haemodynamically unstable patient is as follows:[19]

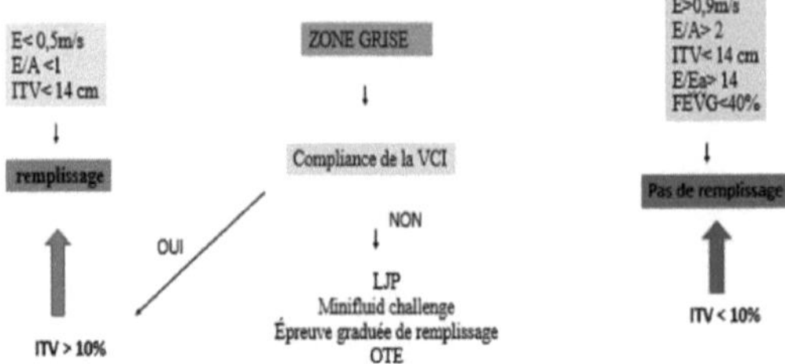


Figure 23: Schema to guide volemic expansion in a patient with haemodynamic instability

Low filling rates associated with a collapsed flow rate are an argument in favour volume expansion.High left filling pressures associated with LV systolic dysfunction are a contraindication to filling.When you find yourself in a grey area, you can use a cellar compliance study: A compliant ICV allows volume expansion under control a parallel variation in VTI. A non-compliant IVC requires use of a filling test, a LJP manoeuvre or an OTE to look for a state of dependent preload.

## 5. ASSESSMENT OF VENTRICULAR FUNCTION RIGHT

The aim is to detail the different methods of assessing right ventricular function, diagnose the different aetiologies of this dysfunction and appropriate management[21]. The right ventricle is very sensitive to variations in afterload compared with the left ventricle, so that right-sided flow falls rapidly with a slight increase in right-sided ejection stress. A right ejection defect is accompanied by an increase in LV end-diastolic volume. This excess of right pre-load results in filling at the expense of the left cavities in diastole, prolongation of LV systole time, and another left displacement of the interventricular septum at the time of systole, known as the paradoxical septum, The consequence is a left-sided filling defect and a secondary fall in overall cardiac output, Low left-sided flow increased right-sided ejection stress LV ischaemia, which exacerbates ventricular dysfunction and maintains a circle of alteration in bi-ventricular load and flow conditions.

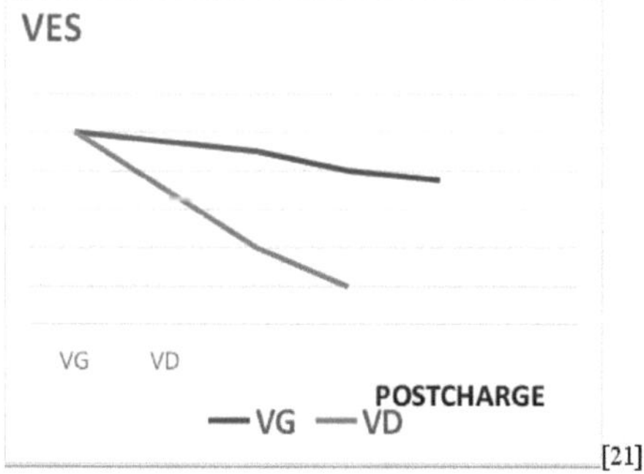


Figure 24: Changes in ESV as a function of ventricular stress level

Lung volumes influence changes in pulmonary vascular resistance. The equilibrium point is represented by the CRF, and any increase in lung volumes is accompanied by an increase in PVRs due to crushing of the intra-alveolar capillary bed. Any decrease in lung volumes leads to an increase in PVR due to crushing of the extra-alveolar capillary bed[22].

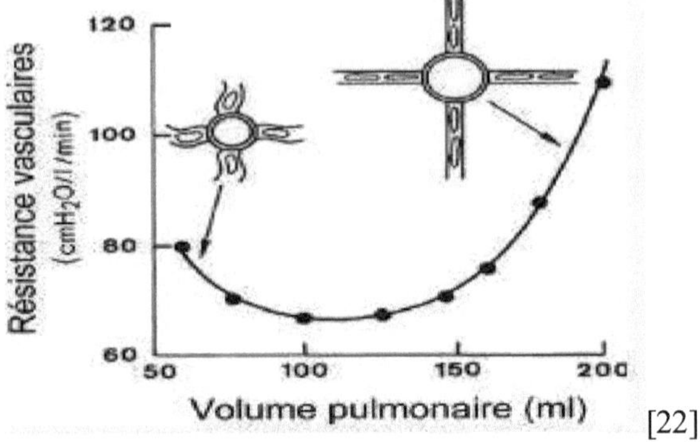

[22]

Figure 25: Changes in pulmonary vascular resistance as a function of lung volumes

## 5.1 MORPHOLOGICAL ANALYSIS OF CAVITIES

Assessment of right ventricular function should begin with an overall morphological analysis, assessment of both systolic and diastolic function, measurement of pulmonary pressures, and end with an investigation of the acute or chronic nature of right ventricular damage if present.[23] This is the first step in the evaluation of right ventricular function. Assessment of the overall morphology requires an approach based on different windows and exploration sections of the right cavities. The apical 4-cavity section measures the VD/VD ratio The parasternal long-axis section is used to measure the VD diameter and the thickness of the VD free wall. The short axis is useful for assessing septal movement and compression and for measuring the diameter of the pulmonary artery.

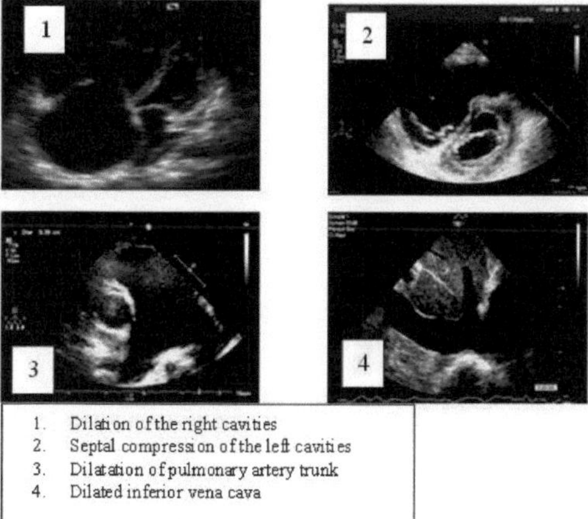


Figure 26: Morphological analysis of the right cavities by echocardiography

## 5.2 EVALUATION OF SYSTOLIC FUNCTION VD

There are not many recommended indices for assessing LV function (the disc method is not indicated because of the complex ventricular architecture).
right[24]) the fraction of VD surface shortening must be greater than 50%.

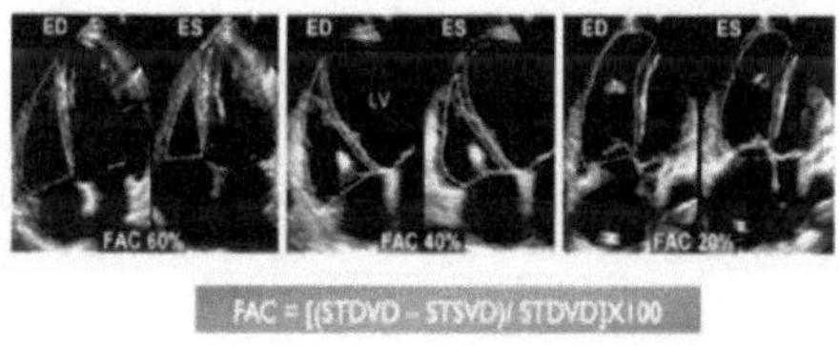


Figure 27: VD surface shortening fraction

Several other indices can be used assess LV systolic function: The degree of displacement of the lateral annulus of the tricuspid valve, known as TAPSE, is equal on average to 24 mm. The speed of movement of the annulus measured in systole by tissue Doppler is pathological if it is less than 9.5 cm/s.

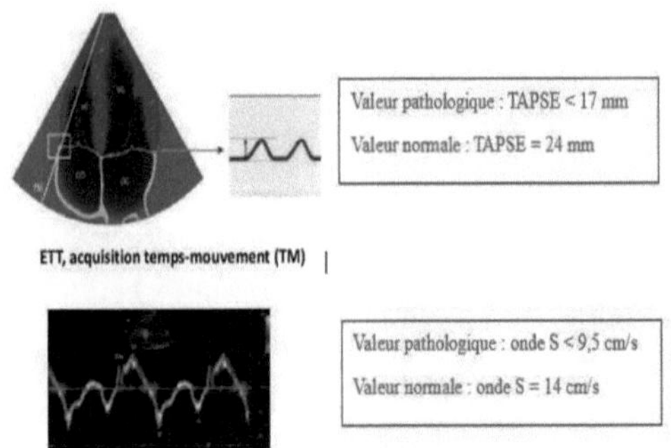


Figure 28: Assessment LV systolic function

The different indices used assess right ventricular systolic function are summarised in Table 1 :

Table 1: Indices used assess systolic VD function

| Assessment criteria | Formulas | Normal values | Pathological values |
|---|---|---|---|
| TAPSE | | 24 mm | < 17 mm |
| FEVD 3D | | 58% | < 45% |
| FRS | STD- STS/STD | 50% | < 35% |
| Tricuspid S-wave | | 14 cm /s | < 9.5 cm /s |

TAPSE: tricuspid annulus systolic excursion. FEVD: LV ejection (MRI). FRS: fraction shortening in surfaces

## 5.3 EVALUATION OF DIASTOLIC FUNCTION VD

Diastolic right ventricular function can be explored from the tricuspid filling flow called the tricuspid profile, the deceleration time of the tricuspid Et wave, and by assessment of LV compliance (Et/Ea t ratio) (Tab 2) [27]

Table 2: Indices assessing LV diastolic function

| Indices | Average values | Pathological values |
|---|---|---|
| Tricuspid TDE | 180 ms | < 120 ms |
| E/Ea tricuspid | 1,4 | > 2 |
| Speed of movement of the lateral ring in diastole | 14 cm /s | < 7.8 cm /s |

The simplest method used in intensive care to assess right pressures is the study of inferior venous compliance, which is an indirect reflection of central venous pressure, which is a poor marker of the state of dependent preload. CVP remains a reliable marker for peripheral organ , particularly renal damage.

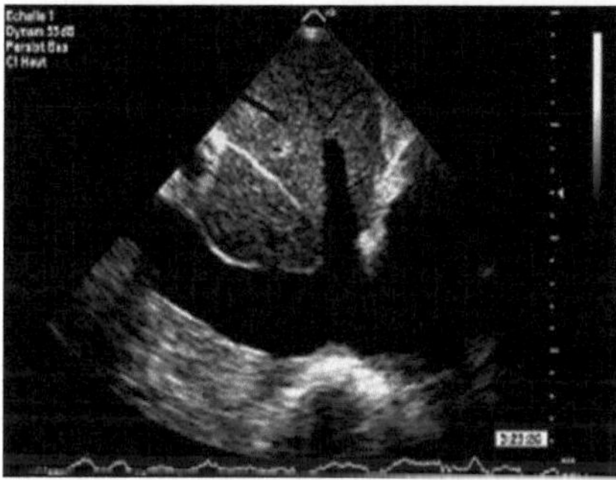

Figure 29: Dilated IVC with high straight filling pressures

The most important aspect of a study of inferior vena cava compliance is the variation in diameter between the inspiratory and expiratory times. Measurement of the max diameter alone does not reflect compliance. +++

### 5.4 ASSESSMENT OF PULMONARY PRESSURES

Pre-capillary pulmonary pressures are assessed using BERNOULLI's physical principle [29].The pressure gradient between two chambers depends on the leakage velocity between the two cavities.Systolic blood pressure (SBP) is calculated from IT leakage velocityDiastolic pulmonary artery pressure (DAPP) and mean pulmonary artery pressure (MAPP) are calculated from the IP leak rate using the same formula.Pulmonary vascular resistance can be measured using the ABBAS formula, which is the ratio of pressure deduced from IT velocity to right-sided flow deduced from pulmonary ITV.

Pulmonary IT/ITV speed

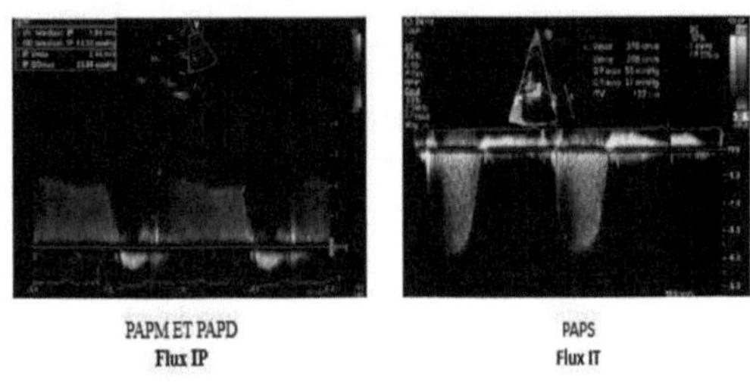


Formule de BERNOULLI : DELTA P = 4 X Vitesse de fuite IT2

Figure 30: Measurement of pulmonary pressures

## 5.5 CPC/CPA DIAGNOSTIC CRITERIA ?

diagnosis of chronic or acute right-sided involvement can be deduced from the clinical context.Elevated pulmonary pressures above 60 mmhg are indicative of chronic right-sided damage, since a previously healthy right ventricle cannot withstand such high ventricular afterload.Finally, dilatation of pulmonary artery trunk is another argument pointing to the chronic nature of the right-sided disease.Table 3 summarises the main parameters used to diagnose between CPC and CPA [23].

Table 3: Clinico-radiological criteria for CPC/CPA referral

| | Acute pulmonary heart disease | Chronic pulmonary heart disease |
|---|---|---|
| Causes | Pulmonary embolism | Chronic respiratory insufficiency, scleroderma, anorectics... |
| Direct signs | VD/VG ratio> 0.6 Non-dilated AP trunk PAPS< 60 mmhg | VD/VG ratio > 1 Dilatation of the AP common trunk PAPS> 60 mmhg |

The aetiologies of right ventricular dysfunction in intensive care are mainly dominated acute obstruction by cruciate emboli (pulmonary embolism), the incidence of which can be as high as 50% (5% of these emboli progress to cardiogenic shock, with a mortality rate that can be as high as 50%). ARDS is another aetiology of APC; it is an echocardiographic definition which combines right dilatation, pulmonary hypertension, a paradoxical septum and, finally, a left repercussion expressed by a disorder of LV relaxation. This damage to the VD during ARDS is closely linked to an increase in PVRs caused hypoxemia, mechanical ventilation and, above all, the loss of lung volume. Finally, there are other aetiologies right-sided involvement, above all infarctions of the right heart complicating posterior ACS, and dysfunctions following cardiac and thoracic surgery.Therapeutic management of right-sided damage is aetiological Thrombolysis or embolectomy for cruciate obstructions, revascularisation for right-sided obstructions. coronary obstructions, protective ventilation with the main aim of maintaining a low level plateau pressure and motor pressure in order to reduce VD afterload. The avoidance of aggravating factors (hypoxaemia, hypercapnia and acidosis) and the use of NO is also recommended to reduce this constraint on right ejection. Management of blood volume is very difficult right heart attacks, and ventricular load conditions means first of all reducing postload by the methods already mentioned.Managing right ventricular preload is not . The right ventricle must not be too full or too empty.

VD volume overload or VD congestion assessed by echocardiography often requires diuretic depletion.

The main objective of the decision to fill a dysfunctional VD is to increase cardiac output by improving the filling of the left cavities.

The dynamic methods used to assess the state of pre-load dependence are not valid in cases of right ventricular dysfunction. This filling is indicated above all in cases where the afterload is not too high.

The introduction a positive inotropic agent is based primarily on the existence echocardiographically documented systolic dysfunction.

Dobutamine improves contractility at the expense tachycardia, which increases energy requirements, and hypotension, which alters coronary perfusion pressure.

**Noradrenaline** is the best agent used in right ventricular pharmacological assistance, improving contractility and coronary perfusion pressure without much energy expenditure and without significantly increasing pulmonary vascular resistance if the dose used is less than 0.5 gamma/kg/min.

## 6. PERICARDIAL EFFUSIONS

Pericarditis is defined as an inflammatory reaction of the pericardial sac. The presence a liquid pericardial effusion in an inflammatory pericardial reaction is not constant.The presence a fluid effusion in the pericardial sac is not always secondary to an inflammatory reaction and does not mean pericarditis. The element to be feared in a pericardial effusion is the compression of the cardiac chambers producing a state of pre-tamponade or tamponade [30][31].

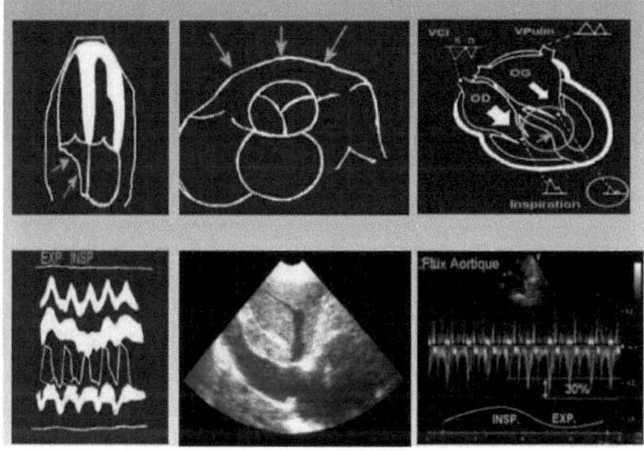


Figure 31: Pericardial fluid effusion, impact on ventricular filling conditions

The first sign of compression will be seen in straight cavities, as these are low-pressure cavities.Invagination of the free wall of the right atrium and compression of the VD free wall in diastole are the first signs of poor tolerance of a pericardial effusion. The displacement of the interventricular septum and the compression of the LV in diastole (filling of the right cavities at the expense of the left cavities) leads to a lack of LV filling and a secondary decrease in cardiac output during inspiration, known as Kusmaul's paradoxical pulse. The impact on bi-ventricular filling rates is a logical consequence of a change in myocardial loading conditions (preload and afterload).Cardiac output drops during inspiration and becomes normal expiration Impaired compliance of both vena cava can explained by increased right-sided filling pressures. The patient can defend himself by ventricular systole, which maintains the hollow "x" reflecting the intra-atrial depression, allowing venous return to the right cavities to be maintained. Treatment is straightforward, with evacuation of the effusion by simple puncture improving the patient's clinical situation and the elastance of the ventricular walls, whatever the aetiology of the pericardial effusion.

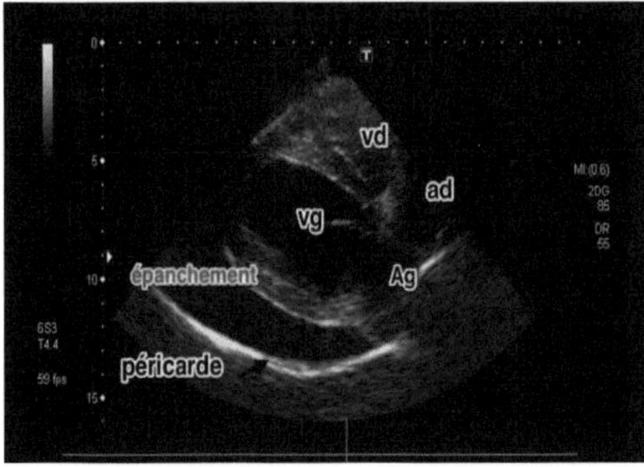


Figure 32: Pericardial fluid effusion

# 7. BIBLIOGRAPHY

1. Gardin JM et al. Recommendations for a standardized report for adult transthoracic echocardiography: a report from the American Society of Echocardiography's Nomenclature and Standards Committee and Task Force for a Standardized Echocardiography Report. J Am Soc Echocardiogr. 2002 Mar;15(3):275-90.

2. Schiller N et al. Recommendations for quantitation of the left ventricle by two-dimensional echocardiography. American Society of Echocardiography Committee on Standards, Subcommittee on Quantitation of Two-Dimensional Echocardiograms. J Am Soc Echocardiogr. 1989 Sep-Oct;2(5):358- 67.

3. Lafitte S et al. Improved reliability for echocardiographic measurement of left ventricular volume using harmonic power imaging mode combined with contrast agent. Am J Cardiol. 2000 May 15;85(10):1234- 8.

4. Uematsu M et al. Myocardial velocity gradient as a new indicator of regional left ventricular contraction: detection by a two-dimensional tissue Doppler imaging technique. J Am Coll Cardiol. 1995 Jul;26(1):217-23.

5. Dumesnil JG et al [Myocardial thickening: a valid parameter in appreciating regional left ventricular function. An electrocardiographic study]. Ann Cardiol Angeiol (Paris). 1975 Nov-Dec;24(6):491-8.

6. Brutsaert, J Am Coll Cardiol, 1993;22(1):318-25 - Vignon P et al. Echocardiographie- Doppler en réanimation. Elservier 2002.

7. Appleton CP et al. Demonstration of restrictive ventricular physiology by Doppler echocardiography. J Am Coll Cardiol. 1988 Apr;11(4):757-68. - Pinamonti B et al. Persistence of restrictive left ventricular filling pattern in dilated cardiomyopathy: an ominous prognostic sign. J Am Coll Cardiol. 1997 Mar 1;29(3):604-12.

8. Sohn DW et al. Assessment of mitral annulus velocity by Doppler tissue

imaging in the evaluation of left ventricular diastolic function. J Am Coll Cardiol. 1997 Aug;30(2):474- 80.
9. Flux de propagation TM couleur - Brun P et al. Left ventricular flow propagation during early filling is related to wall relaxation: a color M-mode Doppler analysis. J Am Coll Cardiol. 1992 Aug;20(2):420-32.
10. ROSSVOLL O et al. Pulmonary venous flow velocities recorded by transthoraci Doppler ultrasound: relation to left ventricular diastolic pressures. J Am Coll Cardio 1993 ;21 :1687- 96.
11. S. Lafitte, M. Lafitte, R. Roudaut. Echocardio-doppler, diastolic function, combined indices. Bordeaux, 2011.
12. SF Nagueh. JASE 2016 ;29 :277-314.
13. Maurizio Cecconi , Christoph Hofer, Jean-Louis Teboul Fluid challenges in intensive care: the FENICE study: A global inception cohort study PMID: 26162676PMCID: PMC4550653 DOI: 10.1007/s00134-015-3850-x
14. C. Roger,L. Zieleskiewicz, C. Demattei, et al. Temporal evolution of fluid in sepsis: the FCREV (Fluid Challenge Revisiting) study. PMID: 31097012. DOI : 10.1186/s13054-019-2448-z
15. J.-L. Teboul. SRLF expert recommendations: "Vascular filling indicators in circulatory failure" doi: 10.1016/j.annfar.2005.04.003
16. Charbonneau H, Riu B, Faron, et al. Predicting preload responsiveness using simultaneous recordings of inferior and superior vena cavae diameters. Crit Care 18: 473. MID: 25189403 PMC4175634 DOI : 10.1186/s13054-014-0473-5
17. A. Caillard, A. Tantot, H. Nougué, Heart-lung interactions SFAR 2014
18. Costachescu T, Denault A, Guimond JG, et al. The hemodynamically unstable patient in the intensive care unit: hemodynamic vs. transesophageal echocardiographic monitoring. Crit Care Med 2002;30:1214-23.
19. L. Muller. Can we really assess patients' blood volume? SFAR 2022 congress

20. Human physiology, Lauralee Sherwood, (ISBN 9782804149130)
21. Stephanazzi J, Guidon-Attali C, Escarment J (1997) Fonction ventriculaire droite : bases physiologiques et physiopathologiques. Ann Fr Anesth Reanim 16:165-86
22. Weber KT, Janicki JS, Shroff SG, et al (1983) The right ventricle: physiologic and pathophysiologic considerations. Crit Care Med 11:323-8
23. Ariel Cohen, Laurie Soulat-Dufour. Echocardiographie_en_pratique. Publisher Lavoisier Medecine Sciences, 2017
24. Rudski LG, Lai WW, Afilalo J et al. Guidelines for the echocardiographic assessment of the right heart in adults: a report from the American Society of Echocardiography endorsed by the European Association of Echocardiography, a registered branch of the European Society of Cardiology, and the Canadian Society of Echocardiography. J Am Soc Echocardiogr, 2010;23:685-713; quiz 786-788.
25. Kukulski T, Hübbert L, Arnold M et al. Normal regional right ventricular function and its change with age: a Doppler myocardial imaging study. J Am Soc Echocardiogr, 2000;13:194-204.
26. Mor-Avi V, Lang RM, Badano LP et al. Current and evolving echocardiographic techniques for the quantitative evaluation of cardiac mechanics: ASE/EAE consensus statement on methodology and indications endorsed by the Japanese Society of Echocardiography. Eur J Echocardiogr, 2011;12:167-205.
27. Klein AL, Leung DY, Murray RD et al. Effects of age and physiologic variables on right ventricular filling dynamics in normal subjects. Am J Cardiol, 1999; 84:440-448.
28. Kircher BJ, Himelman RB, Schiller NB. Noninvasive estimation of right atrial pressure from the inspiratory collapse of the inferior vena cava. Am J Cardiol 1990;66:483-96.

29. Galie, N., Hoeper, M. M., Humbert,, J. A., & Gomez-Sanchez, M. A. (2009). Guidelines for the diagnosis and treatment of pulmonary hypertension: the Task Force for the Diagnosis and Treatment of Pulmonary Hypertension of the European Society of Cardiology (ESC) and the European Respiratory Society (ERS), endorsed by the International Society of Heart and Lung Transplantation (ISHLT). European heart journal, 30(20), 2493-2537.
30. - Schiller NB, Botvinick EH. Right ventricular compression as a sign of cardiac tamponade. Circulation 1977 ;56 :774-9.
31. Merce J, Sagrista-Sauleda J, Permanyer-Miralda G et al. Correlation between clinical and Doppler echocardiographic findings in patients with moderate and large pericardial effusion. Implications for the diagnosis of cardiac tamponade. Am Heart J 1999 ;138 :759-64.
32. - Horowitz MS, Schultz CS, Stinson EB et al. Sensitivity and specificity of echocardiographic diagnosis of pericardial effusion. Circulation 1974 ;50 :239-47

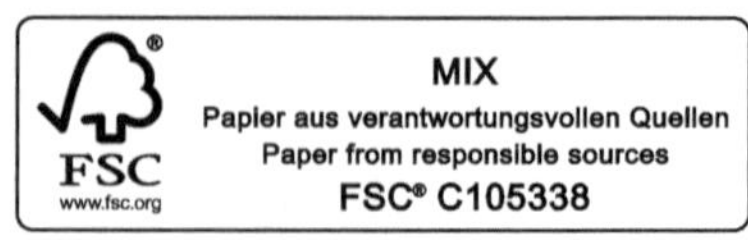


Printed by Books on Demand GmbH, Norderstedt / Germany